CLINICAL PSYCHOPHARMACOLOGY

made
ridiculously
simple

John Preston, Psy.D.
Assistant Professor
Department of Psychiatry
University of California, Davis
School of Medicine

Professional School of Psychology
San Francisco, California

James Johnson, M.D.
Kaiser Medical Center
Department of Psychiatry
South Sacramento, California

ISBN #0-940780-15-1

Made in the United States of America

Published by
MedMaster, Inc.
P.O. Box 640028
Miami, Fla. 33164

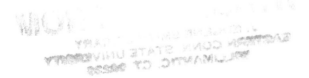

For Bonnie and Mary

Contents

Preface vii

Chapter 1   General Principles 1

Chapter 2   Depression 2

Chapter 3   Bipolar Illness 13

Chapter 4   Anxiety Disorders 19

Chapter 5   Psychotic Disorders 29

Chapter 6   Miscellaneous Disorders 38

Appendix A   History and Personal Data Questionnaire 41

Appendix B   Special Cautions When Taking MAO Inhibitors 43

References 45

Preface

This brief book provides an overview of clinical psychopharmacology. Successful medical treatment of emotional and mental disorders depends on two factors: a thorough knowledge of psychotropic medications and an accurate diagnosis. Both issues are addressed in this book in a practical and concise format.

To the best of our knowledge, recommended doses for medications listed in this book are accurate. However, they are not meant to serve as a guide for prescription of medications. Physicians, please check the manufacturer's product information sheet or the *Physicians' Desk Reference* for any changes in dosage schedule or contraindications.

We wish to express our appreciation to the following people who have reviewed this book and made a number of helpful suggestions: John H. Greist, M.D., Donald Klein, M.D., and Patrick Donlon, M.D. Many thanks to Laurie Zenobia for her help in the preparation of the manuscript and to our editor, Dr. Stephen Goldberg, for many helpful suggestions. Finally, special thanks to the staff of the South Sacramento Kaiser, Department of Psychiatry.

Chapter 1   General Principles

BIOLOGY vs. PSYCHOLOGY

For many years a debate raged in psychiatry with regard to the etiology and treatment of major mental disorders. Two opposing camps emerged: biological psychiatry, whose devotees held that psychiatric disorders had an organic basis; and psychologically oriented psychiatry, probably best represented by the psychodynamic movement, whose converts focused on the role of current emotional stressors, early childhood traumas, interpersonal problems, and intrapsychic conflict as causal agents in the development of psychiatric symptomatology. Although these polar views still exist, in recent years there has been an emerging view that encompasses both psychological and physiological factors in the etiology and treatment of many psychiatric disorders. In many, if not most, mental disorders it is helpful to think of a continuum or spectrum. Almost all mental disorders usually represent rather heterogeneous syndromes.

When one talks about depression, for instance, it is important to realize that depression can present in a number of different ways and may have diverse etiologies. In some instances the cause may be purely psychological, e.g., a reaction to losing a job, death of a loved one, a significant rejection, etc. Likewise, symptoms may be largely psychological, e.g., feelings of low self-esteem and sadness. In other cases the picture is one of a pure biological disorder which has little or no connection to environmental precipitants, but rather involves an endogenous neurochemical malfunction. In addition to psychological symptoms, the resulting symptoms may include a host of somatic symptoms, such as sleep disturbance and weight loss. Clearly, in some individuals there is an interplay of environmental/psychological factors *and* biochemical dysfunctions. The question "Is this a psychological or biological problem?" is overly simplistic. Rather, one must ask, "To what extent is this disorder due to psychological factors and to what extent is it due to a biochemical disturbance?" The answer to this question is extremely important in guiding treatment decisions. *Most purely psychological problems are not helped by medication treatment. On the other hand, most biologically based psychiatric disorders require medication treatment.*

In this book we hope to provide key diagnostic guidelines to help the clinician pinpoint the diagnosis and develop a realistic treatment plan.

Chapter 2   Depression

DIAGNOSIS

Major Clinical Features and Differential Diagnosis

It is important to distinguish between (1) reactive sadness, (2) grief, (3) medical illness and medications that cause depressive symptoms, and (4) clinical depression. The first two are painful but normal emotional reactions and usually do not require treatment. These four syndromes may be distinguished by the following characteristics:

1. *Reactive Sadness* The emotional reaction stems from a relatively minor event. It is transient (a few hours to a few days) and rarely interferes with functioning.

2. *Grief.* This is a normal response to a major interpersonal loss (such as the death of a loved one or marital separation/divorce). This process can be tremendously painful and is much more prolonged then reactive sadness. Grief differs from clinical depression in three ways:

   a. Despite intense sadness, there is no significant loss of self-esteem.

   b. The patient clearly relates the sadness to the loss. There may be active mourning and pining for the loved one; the painful feelings "make sense."

   c. Time is often the major ingredient necessary for emotional healing.

3. *Medical Illnesses and Medications That Can Cause Depression.* Certain medical disorders (see Figure 1) can at times result in biochemical changes that affect central neurotransmitters, thereby triggering serious depressive reactions. Likewise, some medications can cause depression as a side effect (see Figure 2). Please note that minor tranquilizers may cause or exacerbate depression by depleting serotonin, which is a key neurotransmitter implicated in some types of depression. A very frequent treatment mistake is for the physician to be impressed by the more obvious symptoms of anxiety or agitation, to fail to recognize an underlying depression, and to prescribe a benzodiazepine/minor tranquilizer. The result is often some initial calming, but after a week or two the depression worsens. If the basic disorder is depression, but with coexisting anxiety symptoms, it is important to treat the

2

depression. With appropriate treatment for the depression, the anxiety symptoms will subside.

When the basic cause of depression is one of the illnesses listed in Figure 1 or a side effect of medication, the primary focus should be on treating the core illness or switching medications. When such interventions are carried out, the depression will usually lift.

Figure 1

COMMON DISORDERS THAN CAN CAUSE DEPRESSION

Addison's disease

AIDS

Asthma

Chronic infection (mononucleosis, TB)

Congestive heart failure

Cushing's disease

Diabetes

Hyperthyroidism

Hypothyroidism

Infectious Hepatitis

Influenza

■ Malignancies (cancer)

■ Malnutrition

■ Anemia

■ Multiple sclerosis

■ Prophyria

■ Premenstrual syndrome

■ Rheumatoid arthritis

■ Syphilis

■ Systemic lupus erythematosis

■ Uremia

■ Ulcerative colitis

4. *Clinical Depression.* This is a pathological process characterized as follows:

   a. Depressed mood (sadness or emptiness) is often continuous and pervasive.

   b. There is increasing impairment of normal functioning (work, school, and intimate relationships).

   c. There is an irrational or exaggerated erosion of self-esteem.

   d. There is a dramatic and specific change in vegetative patterns (e.g., sleep, appetite, sex drive, etc.) and the appearance of nonspecific physical complaints.

   e. In contrast to grief, the patient is often puzzled as to why he is depressed.

Figure 2

DRUGS THAT MAY CAUSE DEPRESSION

TYPE	GENERIC NAME	BRAND NAME
Antihypertensives (for high blood pressure)	reserpine	Serpasil, Ser-Ap-Es, Sandril
	propranolol hydrochloride	Inderal
	methyldopa	Aldomet
	guanethidine sulfate	Ismelin sulfate
	clonidine hydrochloride	Catapres
	hydralazine hydrochloride	Apresoline hydrochloride
Corticosteroids and other Hormones	cortisone acetate	Cortone
	estrogen	Evex, Menrium, Femest
	progesterone	Lipo-Lutin, Progestasert, Proluton
Antiparkinson Drugs	levodopa and carbidopa	Sinemet
	levodopa	Dopar, Larodopa
	amantadine hydrocholoride	Symmetrel
Antianxiety Drugs	diazepam	Valium
	chlordiazepoxide	Librium
Birth Control Pills	progesterone estrogen	Various Brands
Alcohol	wine, beer, spirits	Various Brands

Target Symptoms

All types of depression tend to share certain universal symptoms (see Figure 3). Disorders that reflect a basic biochemical dysfunction present with *both* the universal symptoms *and* the physiological symptoms, listed below: (See Figure 4.)

Figure 3

SYMPTOMS COMMON TO ALL DEPRESSIONS

■ Mood of sadness, despair, emptiness

■ Anhedonia (loss of the ability to experience pleasure)[1]

■ Low self-esteem

■ Apathy, low motivation, and social withdrawal

■ Excessive emotional sensitivity

■ Negative, pessimistic thinking

■ Irritability

■ Suicidal ideas

---

[1]*Note:* Some degree of decreased capacity for pleasure may be seen in all types of depression. In depressions that involve a biochemical disturbance, this loss of ability to experience pleasure can become so pronounced that the patient has almost no moments of joy or pleasure. Such people are said to have a "non-reactive mood," which means that they are unable to temporarily get out of their depressed mood.

ANTIDEPRESSANT MEDICATION

When Do You Prescribe Antidepressants?

The most important guideline for prescribing antidepressant medication is whether or not there are sustained physiological symptoms, as outlined below (see Figure 4). Occasional disturbances of sleep or appetite, for instance, do not warrant medication treatment. However, if there is continuing weight loss, marked fatigue each day, and poor sleep most nights, antidepressants are indicated. In the Appendix we have included a brief symptom checklist that can be used to quickly assess a host of psychiatric symptoms. Depressive symptoms are included under Section A.

Choosing Medication

Antidepressant medications fall into two primary groups: (1) heterocyclics, and (2) MAO inhibitors. The choice of medications is determined largely by the side effect profile (see Figure 5). The side effects of antidepressant medications often result in serious compliance problems, although some side effects can at times be clinically useful (e.g., sedation for patients with marked agitation or severe sleep disturbances).

Figure 4

PHYSIOLOGICAL SYMPTOMS REFLECTING A BIOCHEMICAL DYSFUNCTION
(TARGET SYMPTOMS FOR MEDICATION TREATMENT)

- Sleep disturbance (early morning awakening, frequent awakenings throughout the night,[1] occasionally hypersomnia: excessive sleeping)

- Appetite disturbance (decreased or increased, with accompanying weight loss or gain)

- Fatigue

- Decreased sex drive

- Restlessness, agitation, or psychomotor retardation

- Diurnal variations in mood (usually feeling worse in the morning)

- Impaired concentration and forgetfulness

- Pronounced anhedonia (total loss of the ability to experience pleasure)

[1]*Note:* Initial insomnia (difficulty in falling asleep) may be seen with depression but is not diagnostic of a major depressive disorder. Initial insomnia can be seen in anyone experiencing stress in general. Initial insomnia alone is more characteristic of anxiety disorders than of depression.

If medications are indicated, first assess the patient's motor state. An agitated, restless patient may do better with a more sedating antidepressant, and a more lethargic, fatigued patient may do better with a less sedating antidepressant. (See Figure 5).

Second, consider the special problems that the patient may have. Some medications have selective effects. (See Figure 7).

Prescribing Treatment

Antidepressant medications are always started at a low dosage and gradually titrated up. The most common mistake made by family physicians is to undermedicate. Although there are exceptions, generally a patient must receive a dose that is within the therapeutic range (see Figure 5). As an example, a typical start-up regime for desipramine would be 25 mg. qhs for 2 days. This should be

Figure 5

ANTIDEPRESSANT MEDICATIONS

| *NAMES* | | USUAL DAILY DOSAGE | | ACH |
GENERIC	BRAND	RANGE	SEDATION	EFFECTS[1]
HETEROCYCLICS				
imipramine	Tofranil	150–300 mg	mid	mid
desipramine	Norpramin	150–300 mg	low	low
amitriptyline	Elavil	150–300 mg	high	high
nortriptyline	Aventyl, Pamelor	75–125 mg	mid	mid
protriptyline	Vivactil	15–40 mg	low	mid
trimipramine	Surmontil	100–300 mg	high	mid
doxepin	Sinequan, Adapin	150–300 mg	high	mid
maprotiline	Ludiomil	150–225 mg	mid	low
amoxapine	Asendin	150–400 mg	mid	low
trazodone	Desyrel[2]	150–400 mg	mid	none
fluoxetine	Prozac	20–80 mg	low	none
bupropion	Wellbutrin[2]	200–450 mg	low	none
sertraline	Zoloft	50–200 mg	low	none
paroxetine	Paxil	20–50 mg	low	none
venlafaxine	Effexor	75–375 mg	low	none
MAO INHIBITORS[3]				
phenelzine	Nardil	30–90 mg	low	none
tranylcypromine	Parnate	20–60 mg	low	none
isocarboxazid	Marplan	20–40 mg	low	none

[1]*ACH EFFECTS* (anticholinergic side effects) include dry mouth, constipation, difficulty in urinating, and blurry vision. Can cause confusion and memory disturbances in the elderly or brain damaged patient.

[2]Due to short half-life, requires divided dosing.

[3]Require strict adherence to dietary and medication regimen.

Note: prescribe maprotiline and bupropion to patients with history of seizures only with great caution.

increased by 25 mg every 2–3 days as long as side effects are minimal, until the patient reaches a solid therapeutic level, i.e., at least 150 mg q.d. Often it takes from 10–14 days to reach a dosage that is within the therapeutic range. Faster increases often result in side effects and compliance problems. Slower increases prolong the suffering caused by the depression. With selective serotonin re-uptake inhibitors (SSRI's: fluoxetine, sertraline, paroxetine) often the starting dose (20 mg., 50 mg., 20 mg., respectively) is the dose that is therapeutic. Increases in dose can be made if there is a failure to show a positive response after 4–5 weeks of treatment.

What to Expect

Neuro-researchers have hypothesized that many of the primary symptoms of clinical depression are caused by a dysregulation of certain neurotransmitters

Figure 6

DECISION TREE FOR DIAGNOSIS
AND TREATMENT OF DEPRESSION

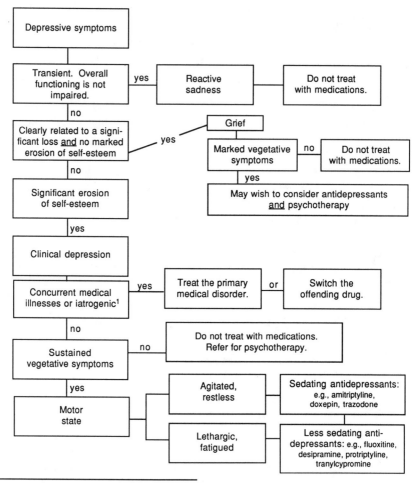

¹ See Figures 2 and 3

(e.g., norepinephrine and serotonin). Antidepressant medications are able to restore normal neuronal functioning in key limbic structures in the brain. It is very important to note, however, that these drugs do not act rapidly. It generally requires 10 to 21 days of treatment for symptoms to start to improve. This is a crucial point. Many, if not most, depressed patients become easily discouraged if there is no relief in a few days. Such patients often discontinue medications prematurely. In prescribing antidepressant medication, patient education is especially important. Listed below are the key points to communicate to patients starting on antidepressants.

Figure 7
SPECIAL PROBLEMS AND MEDICATIONS OF CHOICE

THE PROBLEM	*DRUGS OF CHOICE*
1. High suicide risk[1]	1. trazodone, fluoxetine, sertraline, paroxetine, bupropion
2. Concurrent depression and panic attacks	2. phenelzine, imipramine, fluoxetine
3. Chronic pain with or without depression	3. amitriptyline, doxepin
4. Weight gain on other antidepressants	4. fluoxetine, bupropion, sertraline, paroxetine
5. Sensitivity to anti-cholinergic side effects	5. trazodone, fluoxetine, phenelzine, tranylcypromine, bupropion, sertraline, paroxetine
6. Orthostatic hypotension	6. nortriptyline, bupropion, sertraline

[1]*Note:* Most antidepressants are quite toxic when taken in an overdose. Extreme caution should be exercised in prescribing to high-risk suicidal patients. Of the existing antidepressants, trazodone appears to have the lowest degree of cardiotoxicity.

KEY POINTS TO COMMUNICATE TO PATIENTS

1. Onset of clinical action generally takes 10–21 days. It will take this long for you to notice a reduction of symptoms.

2. Symptomatic improvement is usually seen primarily in the physiological symptoms (Figure 4). Many of the other symptoms (e.g., depressed mood, low self-esteem, etc.) may respond only partially to medication treatment. These medications are not "happy pills"; they do not totally erase feelings of sadness or emptiness.

3. The best barometers of early medication response generally include improved sleep, less daytime fatigue, and some improvement in emotional control (e.g., less frequent crying spells or better frustration tolerance). The physician may need to inquire specifically about these symptoms because many depressed people will say "I'm no better," despite the fact that there is symptomatic improvement.

4. There may be side effects. However, side effects can most often be managed by dosage adjustment or by switching to another medication.

5. Total length of treatment varies considerably for individuals. Typically, it may take 4–8 weeks for the major depressive symptoms to subside. It is very important not to discontinue treatment at this point. The relapse rate can be as high as 80%. The general rule of thumb is to continue treatment for a

9

period of 4–6 months beyond the point of symptomatic improvement and then gradually to reduce the dose. Should symptoms return during this medication-reduction phase of treatment, the dosage should again be increased. Medication should be continued for 4–6 weeks before another trial on lower doses. Occasionally, a person may need to be on long-term, chronic medication management.

6. Antidepressants are not addictive.

7. You should not drink alcohol when taking antidepressants. Alcohol can block the effects of the antidepressants (although, in clinical practice, many physicians will allow patients on antidepressants to have an occasional drink, but not in excess of one per day).

Treatment-Resistant Depressions

Generally it is best to start with a heterocyclic. It is necessary to treat at adequate doses; most treatment failures are due to inadequate doses. Unless side effects are intolerable or a person is a high risk patient (see *Precautions* below), standard practice is to push the dose to the upper level of the therapeutic range until symptomatic improvement is attained. If a patient is on a high dose for a period of 3–4 weeks without symptomatic improvement it is unlikely that improvement will occur. A second strategy that often produces positive results is to add a low dose of lithium (600 to 900 mg. per day) to the antidepressant. A fairly large number of non-respondents do benefit from lithium augmentation (Greist, 1989, personal communication). Should this fail, then a change in the antidepressant medication is in order.

The next step generally is to switch to another heterocyclic. The choice is guided by two factors: side effect profiles and neurotransmitter action. There is some evidence to suggest that there exist two basic neurochemicals that may be affected in major depressive disorder: norepinephrine and serotonin. The various heterocyclic medications have different effects on these two neurochemical systems (see Figure 8). Some are considered to have broad spectrum effects ("shotguns") and others are more selective ("bullets"). The disadvantage in choosing a broad spectrum drug is that they typically have more troublesome side effects. If your first unsuccessful drug was serotonergic, then the second choice should be a medication targeting norepinephrine.

What if this fails too? A fourth strategy is to switch to either bupropion or to an MAO inhibitor. Treatment is described below. The final option is electroconvulsive therapy (ECT) which is a highly effective, albeit costly, form of treatment for depression.

Dysthymia

Dysthymia is a type of mild, chronic depressive disorder characterized by the following symptoms (which are present almost every day over a period of 2+ years):

Figure 8

SELECTIVE ACTION OF ANTIDEPRESSANT MEDICATIONS

GENERIC	BRAND	NOREPINEPHRINE	SEROTONIN	MONOAMINE OXIDASE	DOPAMINE
imipramine	Tofranil	+ +	+ + +	0	0
desipramine	Norpramin	+ + + + +	0	0	0
amitriptyline	Elavil	+	+ + + +	0	0
nortriptyline	Aventyl, Pamelor	+ + +	+ +	0	0
protriptyline	Vivactil[1]	+ + + +	+	0	0
trimipramine	Surmontil[1]	+ +	+ +	0	0
doxepin	Sinequan, Adapin[1]	+ + +	+ +	0	0
maprotiline	Ludiomil	+ + + + +	0	0	0
amoxapine	Asendin	+ + + +	+	0	0
venlafaxine	Effexor	+ +	+ + +	0	+
trazodone	Desyrel	0	+ + + + +	0	0
fluoxetine	Prozac	0	+ + + + +	0	0
paroxetine	Paxil	0	+ + + + +	0	0
sertraline	Zoloft	0	+ + + + +	0	0
bupropion	Wellbutrin[2]	0	0	0	+
phenelzine	Nardil	0	0	+ + + + +	0
tranylcypromine	Parnate	0	0	+ + + + +	0
isocarboxazid	Marplan	0	0	+ + + + +	0

[1]Uncertain, but likely effects.
[2]Atypical antidepressant. Uncertain effects but likely to be a dopamine agonist.

- Daytime fatigue

- Negative, Pessimistic thinking

- Low self-esteem

- Low motivation, low enthusiasm

- Decreased capacity for joy

Evidence from a number of recent studies suggests that 50–55% of patients with dysthymia can respond favorably to a trial on anti-depressant medications.

Precautions: Tricyclic Antidepressants

The following patients should either not be treated or treated cautiously with tricyclics: immediate post-MI patients, epileptics, patients with narrow-angle glaucoma, and pregnant women. The physician should consult package inserts and the *Physicians' Desk Reference* for more details regarding precautions and contraindications.

MAO Inhibitors

Two commonly used MAOI's, phenelzine and tranylcypromine have been shown to be as effective as tricyclics in a number of studies. However, shortly after their introduction into the United States in the 1950's there were reports of severe reactions in some patients, which resulted in great concern in the medical community. The drugs interact with certain medications (sympathomimetic amines) and with certain foods (containing tyramine, a natural byproduct of bacterial fermentation processes, found in many cheeses, some wines and beers, and foods such as chopped liver, broad beans, chocolate, snails, etc.). (See Appendix B.) The interaction resulted in a severe hypertensive crisis, which for a number of patients was fatal. So for many years these medications were abandoned because doctors viewed them as unsafe. However, especially in Europe, doctors recognized that these drugs had clinical utility and could be safely used if certain dietary restrictions were followed. In fact, in Europe during the past 25 years the MAOI's have probably been used as much as the tricyclics.

Just recently the MAOI's have been rediscovered by American medicine and are now enjoying a renaissance for several reasons. First, if dietary restrictions are observed, these drugs are actually safer than the tricyclics and have fewer side effects. Secondly, they have been found to work in many patients who do not respond to tricyclics. And finally, some studies indicate that MAOI's may be the drug of choice for some types of affective disorders including atypical depressions presenting primarily with anxiety and phobic symptoms, masked depressions (e.g., hypochondriasis), and anorexia nervosa.

Otherwise, guidelines for treatment and clinical response are similar to those previously described for the tricyclics. (See pages 5–11.) The one exception is the important dietary/medication restrictions that must be observed (see Appendix B, patient handout for specific restrictions).

Books to Recommend to Patients

1. *You Can Beat Depression: A Guide to Recovery* by John Preston, Psy.D., Impact Publishers, P.O. Box 1094, San Luis Obispo, CA 93406 (1989).

2. *Feeling Good* by David Burns, M.D., New American Library (1980).

3. *Depression and Its Treatment* by John Greist, M.D. and James Jefferson, M.D., Warner Books (1984).

Chapter 3   Bipolar Illness

DIAGNOSIS

Major Clinical Features and Differential Diagnosis

The diagnosis of a bipolar disorder is based on two sources of data: the current clinical picture (depression or mania) and a clear history of both manic and depressive episodes. The depressive episodes may range from minor to major depressive syndromes as outlined in Chapter 2. Manic episodes typically are described as either full blown mania or less intense manic episodes, referred to as hypomania.

It is important to rule out medical causes of bipolar illness. (See Figures 2 and 3 in Chapter 2 and Figures 9 and 10.)

Figure 9

COMMON DISORDERS THAT MAY CAUSE MANIA

- Brain tumors
- CNS syphilis
- Delirium (due to various causes)
- Encephalitis
- Influenza
- Metabolic changes associated with hemodialysis
- Metastatic squamous adenocarcinoma
- Multiple sclerosis
- Q   fever

Figure 10

DRUGS THAT MAY CAUSE MANIA

- amphetamines
- bromides
- cocaine
- isoniazid
- procarbazine
- steroids

Several classification schemes for bipolar disorders have been proposed by various authors. The two most clinically useful classifications are outlined below:

A. *BIPOLAR I* vs. *BIPOLAR II*

1. *Bipolar I* This disorder fits the more classic description of bipolar illness with clearly recognized episodes of depression and mania.

2. *Bipolar II* This disorder presents with obvious episodes of depression; but the manic phases of the illness are often less intense, unrecognized, and thus not reported by the patient. If you inquire about manic episodes, the patient will give the impression that none have occurred. The best ways to diagnose such conditions are either to witness a hypomanic episode clinically or to carefully inquire about the history. In particular, if hypomanic episodes are suspected, the most important question to ask is, "Have you ever had a period of time when you didn't need as much sleep?" A decreased need for sleep and a lack of daytime fatigue are red flags for hypomania.

B. *TYPICAL BIPOLAR* vs. *RAPID CYCLING BIPOLAR DISORDERS*

In the more typical bipolar patient, depressive and manic episodes last for several weeks to several months, often with periods of normal mood occurring between periods of depression and mania. When there are two or more episodes of *both* depression and mania (i.e., depression-mania-depression-mania) within a year, this is referred to as "rapid cycling" (DSM-III-R, 1987, p. 225). Sometimes rapid cyclers can dramatically switch moods from week to week or even day to day.

The subclassifications of Bipolar I vs. Bipolar II and typical vs. rapid cycling are important because they have different treatment implications.

Target Symptoms

The target symptoms vary depending on the current phase of the illness. Major depressive symptoms are listed in Chapter 2 (Figure 4). Manic episodes are identified by the following clinical features:

Figure 11

SYMPTOMS OF MANIA[1]

■ A pronounced and persistent mood of euphoria (elevated or expansive mood) or irritability and at least three of the following:

■ Grandiosity or elevated self-esteem

■ Decreased need for sleep

■ Rapid, pressured speech (Often these people are hard, if not impossible, to interrupt.)

■ Racing thoughts

■ Distractibility

■ Increased activity or psychomotor agitation

■ Behavior that reflects expansiveness (lacking restraint in emotional expression) and poor judgment, such as increased sexual promiscuity, gambling, buying sprees, giving away money, etc.

---

[1]Adapted from DSM-III-R, 1987 (with permission), p. 217. Also see Questions 1–10 and 11–14 on the History and Personal Data Questionnaire (Appendix A.)

MEDICATIONS USED TO TREAT BIPOLAR ILLNESS

When Do You Prescribe Medications?

Treatment of bipolar disorders has two goals. The first goal is the reduction of current symptoms, and the second is the prevention of relapse. Bipolar disorders are invariably recurring and thus prophylactic treatment is warranted.

Choosing Medication

The primary medication used to treat this disorder is lithium. However a number of other drugs have been found to be effective as adjuncts or alternatives to lithium. We will describe standard treatment with lithium and then comment on the role of other medications.

Lithium has two primary effects: It stabilizes mood, and in many instances it can prevent relapse (or at least lessen the intensity of subsequent episodes) if treatment is on an ongoing basis. Lithium seems to be somewhat more effective in preventing relapse of mania rather than depression.

Prescribing Treatment

The treatment of bipolar disorders can be quite complex. Generally a referral to a specialist is recommended.

If the presenting phase is a manic episode. Often, especially if the patient is quite agitated, out of control or psychotic, the initial plan is to begin treatment with *both* lithium and an antipsychotic medication. The antipsychotics seem to improve behavioral control more rapidly. With lithium, the patient may require 10 days to show a clinical response. Once mood has been stabilized, the antipsychotic may be phased out.

Treatment is initiated after necessary lab tests are conducted (see Figure 12.) Generally the starting dose is 600 or 900 mg./day. given in divided doses. The therapeutic range and toxic range of lithium are very close to one another. Thus it is necessary to gradually increase the dose while carefully monitoring blood levels. Most patients must reach a level between 1.0 and 1.2 mEq/L. Not infrequently the level may need to be higher to obtain symptomatic improvement (1.2 to 1.6), but on these higher levels, side effects are more common and compliance is poorer. On occasion, patients may need and tolerate blood levels up to 2.0 mEq/L. However, there is increased risk of toxicity at such doses. Generally, daily doses range from 1200–3000 mg. Once mood is adequately stabilized, the dose can be lowered somewhat (0.8—1.0 mEq/L) for maintenance treatment.

If the presenting phase is a depressive episode. Because lithium is less effective as an antidepressant, many times, for a patient seen during a depressive phase, treatment is initiated with an antidepressant in combination with lithium. One risk in administering an antidepressant to a bipolar patient is that the drug may precipitate an acute shift into mania. After the depressive episode has resolved, lithium can be used to prevent relapse. Antidepressant treatment is described in Chapter 2, and lithium treatment is the same as previously outlined for a manic episode.

Side Effects of Lithium and Signs of Toxicity

Major side effects include nausea, diarrhea, vomiting, fine hand tremor, sedation, muscular weakness, polyuria, polydypsia, edema, weight gain and a dry mouth. Adverse effects from chronic use may include leukocytosis (reversible upon discontinuation of lithium), hypothyroidism and goiter, acne, psoriasis,

16

teratogenesis (NOTE: lithium is found in breast milk), nephrogenic diabetes insipidus (reversible), and kidney damage.

Signs of toxicity include lethargy, ataxia, slurred speech, tinnitus, severe nausea/vomiting, tremor, arrhythmias, hypotension, seizures, shock, delirium, coma, and death. Since the toxic range is near to the therapeutic range, blood levels and adverse effects must be monitored closely. In addition, a number of other clinical lab tests should be conducted at the beginning of treatment and periodically thereafter (see Figure 12).

Figure 12

CLINICAL LAB TESTS FOR PATIENTS TAKING LITHIUM

- Na (Sodium)
- Ca (Calcium)
- P (Phosphorus)
- EKG

- Creatinine
- Urinalysis
- Complete CBC
- Thyroid battery (with TSH)

Listed below are the key points that should be communicated to patients starting treatment with lithium.

KEY POINTS TO COMMUNICATE TO PATIENTS

1. Lithium is a medication that treats your current emotional problem and will also be helpful in preventing relapse. So it will be important to continue with treatment after the current episode is resolved.

2. Since the therapeutic and toxic dosage ranges are so close, we must monitor your blood level closely. This will be done more frequently at first and every several months thereafter. Never increase your dose without first consulting with your physician.

3. Lithium is not addictive.

4. Many side effects can be reduced/minimized by taking divided doses or may subside as treatment progresses.

5. Bipolar disorders often run in families. Any relatives that have pronounced mood swings should be alerted to the possibility of a treatable condition and the need for professional evaluation. (The yield on this maneuver is still high, since medical awareness of bipolar disorder is still low, especially with milder forms, and family history is impressively often positive for this disorder.)

6. You and your family need to be aware that this is a biological disorder, not a moral defect or a character flaw. When severe, you may not always be able to control your behavior, necessitating that practical steps be taken to protect all concerned from your judgment during episodes.

7. Many self-help groups have been developed to provide support for bipolar patients and their families. In this community, the local self-help group is _____, and you can find out more information by calling _____.

Specialized Treatments for Subtypes of Bipolar Disorder

In addition to standard lithium treatment, many researchers and clinicians have suggested treatment options for certain bipolar subtypes (see Figure 13).

Figure 13

SPECIALIZED TREATMENTS FOR SUBTYPES OF BIPOLAR DISORDERS

SUBTYPE	*MEDICATION ALTERNATIVES*
Bipolar II	MAO inhibitors
Rapid Cyclers	Carbamazepine (Tegretol)

Books to Recommend to Patients

1. *Mood Swings* by Ronald Fieve, M.D., Bantam Books (1975).

2. *Lithium and Manic Depression: A Guide,* Lithium Information Center, Univ. of Wisconsin (1989).

Chapter 4   Anxiety Disorders

DIAGNOSIS

Major Clinical Features and Differential Diagnosis

Six different anxiety disorders are seen in clinical practice. An accurate diagnosis is important as the treatments vary. There is no one treatment appropriate for all anxiety disorders. It is important to distinguish between the following: (1) generalized anxiety disorder (G.A.D.), (2) stress related anxiety, (3) panic disorder, (4) social phobias, (5) medical illnesses presenting with anxiety symptoms, and (6) anxiety symptoms as a part of a primary mental disorder (e.g., depression, schizophrenia).

Before outlining the main features of each disorder, it is necessary to define two terms: panic attacks and anxiety symptoms. Panic attacks are very brief but extremely intense surges of anxiety. The major differences between a panic attack and more generalized anxiety symptoms are differences in the onset, duration, and intensity. Panic attacks often "come out of the blue" (i.e., not necessarily provoked by stress), they come on suddenly, are *extremely* intense, last from 1–20 minutes, and then subside. The patient feels as if he will actually die or go crazy. We are not talking about uneasiness; we are talking about full-blown panic. The person may continue to feel nervous or upset for several hours, but the attack itself lasts only a matter of minutes. If a patient says, "I've had a continuous panic attack for the past three days," he may be having intense anxiety symptoms, but not a true panic attack. In other anxiety disorders, anxiety symptoms can be very unpleasant, but are much less intense; they also can be prolonged or generalized (i.e., present most of the day and last from days to years). The distinction between "symptoms" and "attacks" is very important when it comes to treatment. Please refer to Figure 14.

The six anxiety syndromes can be distinguished by the following characteristics:

1. *Generalized Anxiety Disorder*. The key here is *long-term*, low level, fairly continuous anxiety. Patients with this disorder *may* have no specific current life stressors. To them, daily living provokes anxiety. Such people are chronic worriers, always "what-if-ing" (e.g., "What if I get fired?" "What if my check bounces?" "What if my wife leaves me?").

Figure 14

SYMPTOMS OF ANXIETY[1]

- Trembling, feeling shaky, restlessness, muscle tension
- Shortness of breath, smothering sensation
- Tachycardia (rapid heartbeat)
- Sweating and cold hands and feet
- Lightheadedness and dizziness
- Paresthesias (tingling of the skin)
- Diarrhea and/or frequent urination
- Feelings of unreality (derealization)
- Initial insomnia (difficulty falling asleep)
- Impaired attention and concentration
- Nervousness, edginess, or tension

---

[1]Adapted from DSM-III-R, 1987 (with permission), p. 253

2. *Stress-related Anxiety.* The patient with this disorder typically functions well. However, the anxiety symptoms have recently emerged in the face of major life stresses (e.g., a serious family illness, a marital separation, etc.).

3. *Panic Disorder.* This is characterized by repeated episodes of full-blown panic, as described in the discussion of panic attacks.

4. *Social Phobias.* Anxiety is experienced only when the person is in social/ interpersonal settings, e.g., public speaking, asking someone out for a date, social gatherings.

5. *Medical Illnesses, and Medications Presenting with Anxiety Symptoms.* Certain diseases/conditions can at times result in biochemical changes that produce anxiety symptoms. If someone complains of nervousness or anxiety, it should never be assumed that it is simply an emotional disorder until medical causes have been ruled out (Figure 15). Likewise, a number of medications and over-the-counter products can cause pronounced anxiety symptoms (Figure 16).

Figure 15

COMMON DISORDERS THAT ARE ASSOCIATED WITH ANXIETY

Adrenal tumor

Alcoholism

CNS degenerative diseases

Cushing's disease

Coronary insufficiency

Delirium[1]

Hypoglycemia

■ Hyperthyroidism

■ Meniere's disease (early stages)

■ Parathyroid disease

■ Post-concussion syndrome

■ Premenstrual syndrome

■ Mitral valve prolapse[2]

[1]Delirium can occur as a result of many toxic/metabolic conditions and often produces anxiety and agitation.
[2]The mitral valve prolapse probably does not cause anxiety, but it has been found that MVP and anxiety disorders often coexist. This may be due to some underlying common genetic factor.

Figure 16

DRUGS THAT MAY CAUSE ANXIETY

■ Amphetamines

■ Asthma medications

■ Caffeine

■ CNS depressants (withdrawal)

■ Cocaine

■ Nasal decongestant sprays

■ Steroids

6. *Anxiety as a Part of a Primary Mental Disorder.* Anxiety frequently accompanies many mental disorders (e.g., depression, schizophrenia, organic brain syndromes, substance abuse).

ANTIANXIETY MEDICATION * TREATMENT

When Do You Prescribe Antianxiety Medications?

Treatment differs depending on the diagnosis, so each disorder will be addressed separately.

1. *Generalized anxiety disorder (G.A.D.)*. Many physicians have tried to treat this disorder with benzodiazepines. This presents two problems: (1) In the long run, such treatment is often not very effective. (2) Patients can develop tolerance/dependence problems with chronic benzodiazepine use. Many clinicians think that G.A.D. is primarily a psychological (not biological) disorder and recommend psychotherapy. However, recently a new drug, buspirone hydrochloride, has been shown to be effective in treating some G.A.D. patients. An added feature of this medication is that patients do not develop dependence or tolerance. Other minor tranquilizers are usually not indicated in the treatment of G.A.D.

2. *Stress-related anxiety*. Minor tranquilizers are very helpful in reducing anxiety symptoms (especially insomnia and restlessness) which accompany acute situational stress. The most important issue to consider is whether or not the stress is acute and likely to be of short duration. Antianxiety medications should only be used for a period of 1–4 weeks. If it is clear that this is just one in a series of chronic life crises, it is probably best not to prescribe benzodiazepines.

3. *Panic disorder*. One isolated panic attack is generally insufficient evidence of true panic disorder. However, four or more true attacks within a period of one month suggest panic disorder. Look for spontaneous attacks (most "come out of the blue") and episodes that last a matter of minutes (not hours or days). Many patients with other types of disorders say they have panic attacks but on closer inspection, many do not.

4. *Social phobias*. Generally social phobias are not treated medically but with psychotherapy and behavioral approaches. In some cases beta blockers or MAO inhibitors have been helpful.

5. *Medical illnesses/medications causing anxiety symptoms*. In almost all instances, the treatment of choice is to treat the primary medical illness or to discontinue the offending drug. Be cautious in stopping certain drugs; for instance, if a patient stops drinking coffee abruptly, he may have significant withdrawal symptoms which mimic anxiety. Such drugs must be gradually withdrawn.

6. *Anxiety symptoms as a part of another primary mental disorder*. Treat the primary disorder. Minor tranquilizers are usually not indicated.

---

*Also referred to as minor tranquilizers, anxiolytics, and benzodiazepines. These terms will be used interchangeably.

Choosing a Medication

Antianxiety medications fall into five groups (see Figure 17). The primary choice of medication is based on the diagnosis. Secondarily, one should consider certain problematic side effects such as sedation and rapidity of absorption (rapid absorption may be associated with a euphoric "rush").

Prescribing Treatment

1. *Generalized Anxiety Disorder.* Buspirone is the medication of choice. Unlike the benzodiazepines, buspirone is slow acting. It often requires 2–6 weeks of treatment before symptomatic improvement. The major problem encountered with this medication is premature discontinuation by the patient. Patients often expect quick results from medications. It is important to educate the patient about onset of action. Buspirone can be effective in treating many symptoms of G.A.D., but it does not seem to decrease panic attacks. Buspirone must be taken every day; it is not a medication that is taken only when the patient feels anxious. If patients fail to respond to buspirone, if symptoms are severe, and if there is no history of alcohol or other substance abuse, benzodiazepines can be used to treat G.A.D.

2. *Stress-Related Anxiety.* All benzodiazepines are effective in treating acute stress-induced anxiety. (See Figure 17). The most important considerations in choosing a medication have to do with side effects and medication halflife. The most common side effect is sedation. Intense restlessness or agitation may require a more sedating drug; however, in most instances it is better to use low sedation benzodiazepines to reduce daytime anxiety. Of course many anxious patients will present with a sleep disturbance. Insomnia will be addressed below. A second side effect is the so-called euphoric "rush" secondary to the peak in blood level of medication. Such a peak creates a good deal of sedation and can be useful if the goal is to induce sleep, but the euphoric experience can lead to abuse. In addiction-prone individuals it is best to choose a drug that avoids or minimizes this effect. Finally the half life of a medication is an important variable when it comes to discontinuing the drug. Those medications listed that have a shorter half life may need to be discontinued very gradually so as to avoid withdrawal symptoms.

    Dosage ranges vary widely as seen in Figure 17. However, a typical starting dose of lorazepam, for instance, is 0.5 mg. b.i.d. or t.i.d. Such a dose should be increased every three days as needed until a final range of 2–6 mg./day is achieved. The goal is to provide some symptomatic relief over a period of from 1–4 weeks. Should a person still experience significant anxiety after this period of time, a reassessment of the diagnosis is in order.

    It has long been held that long term use of benzodiazepines is contraindicated. Although this is often true, it is not always the case. Recent investigations into chronic benzodiazepine use have shed new light on this clinical practice. Uhlenhuth, et al. (1988, p. 161) report that ". . . many patients continue to derive benefit from long-term treatment with benzodiazepines; and . . . attitudes strongly against the use of these drugs may be depriving

Figure 17

ANTIANXIETY MEDICATIONS

Disorder	Medication Generic	Brand	Usual Daily Dosage Range	Rapidity of Absorption	1/2 life (Hours)
1. G.A.D.	buspirone	BuSpar	5–40 mg.	+	2–8
2. Stress-Related Anxiety	diazepam	Valium	5–40 mg.	+++++	20–50
	chlordiazepoxide	Librium	15–100 mg.	+++	5–30
	oxazepam	Serax	30–120 mg.	++	5–20
	clorazepate	Tranxene	15–60 mg.	++++	30–100
	lorazepam	Ativan	2–6 mg.	+++	10–15
	prazepam	Centrax	20–60 mg.	+	30–100
	alprazolam	Xanax	.25–4 mg.	+++	6–20
	clonazepam	Klonopin	.5–4 mg.	+	80
3. Panic Disorder	alprazolam	Xanax	.25–8 mg.	+++	6–20
	clonazepam	Klonopin	.5–4 mg.	+	80
	tricyclic antidepressants[1]				
	MAO Inhibitors[1]				
4. Social Phobia	propranolol	Inderal	20–80 mg.		
	MAO Inhibitors[1]				
5. Stress-Related Initial Insomnia[2]	flurazepam	Dalmane	15–30 mg.	+++++	40–250[3]
	temazepam	Restoril	15–30 mg.	+++++	10–20
	triazolam	Halcion	.25–.5 mg.	+++++	2–3
	quazepam	Doral	7.5–15 mg.	+++++	39
	zolpidem	Ambien	5–10 mg.	+++++	2–3
	estazolam	Prosom	2–4 mg.	+++++	10–24

[1]See Chapter 2, Figure 5.
[2]Initial insomnia: difficulty falling asleep
[3]Active metabolite (norflurazepam)

many anxious patients of appropriate treatment." The key is to monitor closely for signs of increasing dosage, especially as the patient may be increasing the dosage without medical advice. If in doubt, don't hesitate to get a blood level and to share your concerns openly with the patient. Addiction to benzodiazepines that arise in the course of the treatment of anxiety should be treated for what it is: an occasional and serious side effect. *Always* discontinue benzodiazepines gradually (e.g. if the patient takes 1.5 mg. of alprazolam, q.d., the dose should be reduced by 0.5 mg. per day, per week. This slow taper is especially important with short half-life benzodiazepines).

3. *Stress-Induced Insomnia.* Benzodiazepine sedative-hypnotics can be a safe and efficient treatment for transient initial insomnia. (Recall that middle insomnia and early morning awakening are more indicative of depression and therefore should not be treated with benzodiazepines). Again, in most cases treatment is initiated only if the insomnia is precipitated by recent environmental stress and is not a chronic problem. Chronic insomnia is extremely hard to treat. Note that the newer drug zolpidem tartrate is not a benzodiazepine and studies to-date show that dependence does not occur on this medication. For this reason, it may be a safer alternative in individuals with a substance abuse history. Typical dosages for the various sedatives are listed in Figure 17.

4. *Panic Disorder.* The treatment of panic disorder has two discrete phases.

   Phase One: Eliminate or reduce the frequency or intensity of the panic attacks with antipanic drugs. There are three main groups of antipanic drugs. Let's discuss the pros and cons of each.

   a. High potency benzodiazepines and like compounds (e.g. alprazolam and clonazepam)

      Pros. Very effective. It works quickly, often within days. It also reduces anticipatory anxiety.

      Cons. Although some patients respond to low doses (0.25 mg. t.i.d.), most require much larger doses (3–8 mg/day for alprazolam, 2–4 mg/day for clonazepam), and at these higher doses, sedation is a very common problem. With prolonged use, tolerance can develop. *Very* gradual discontinuation is required to avoid withdrawal symptoms.

   b. Antidepressants: tricyclics and selective serotonin re-uptake inhibitors (SSRIs)

      Pros. Effective in reducing attacks. Can treat concurrent depression. Can be used for prolonged periods of time without risk of tolerance/dependence.

      Cons. Side effects (see Chapter 2) and delayed onset of action (2–3 weeks before symptomatic improvement). Treat in the same way and same dosage levels as you would use to treat depression. Some patients experience an initial increase in panic attacks; these are usually managed well with short term use of lorazepam as necessary. (Note: bupropion is one antidepressant that apparently is not effective in treating panic attacks).

   c. MAO Inhibitors

      Pros. Very effective. Can treat concurrent depression. Can be used for prolonged periods of time without risk of tolerance/dependence.

      Cons. Delayed onset of action (2–3 weeks) and medication/dietary restrictions as outlined in Chapter 2. As with the tricyclics, treat as you would treat depression.

Phase Two. Patients not only have the attacks, but develop significant anticipatory anxiety and avoidance (a strong urge to avoid situations in which they have experienced prior panic attacks, e.g., to avoid crowded stores or driving on freeways). These problems frequently do not spontaneously remit when the panic attacks are eliminated. People continue to have intense worries that "It could happen again." Phase two involves gradual reexposure to feared situations. So if a person is afraid of having an attack at the grocery store, he must gradually approach the feared situation. Only by repeated exposure to the situation and by a series of experiences without panic will the patient's anticipatory anxiety and avoidance diminish. The keys to successful graded reexposure are (1) to effectively control or reduce attacks with medication, and then (2) to have the patient very gradually face the phobic situation.

The duration of the underlying biochemical dysfunction is quite variable. Some people may be treated medically for six months and gradually withdrawn from medication. Others may need years of continued treatment. Like depression, the strategy with any of the antipanic drugs, is to achieve symptomatic relief and then continue to treat for 4–6 months. At that point, a medication-reduction trial may be initiated. If necessary, treatment can be resumed if panic symptoms reemerge.

5. *Social Phobias*. In most cases psychotherapy is the treatment of choice. Psychotropic medications have been used, however, in two types of social phobia. Some social phobics are extremely sensitive to rejection and this is why they are fearful of social interactions. Some new research and clinical data indicate that these patients may benefit from MAO inhibitors. A second type of social phobia, stage fright/public speaking phobia has been successfully treated by beta blockers such as propranolol (usually 20–40 mg., 1 hour prior to performing). Beta blockers do not eliminate the centrally mediated, subjective sense of anxiety, but do quite effectively reduce many peripheral somatic symptoms of anxiety, e.g., tachycardia.

IN EVERY CASE, REMEMBER
Some degree of stress and anxiety is a common part of normal, daily living. Medication treatment should only be initiated if symptoms are significantly intense and severely interfere with normal functioning.
When you prescribe any kind of medication to control anxiety, it is essential to discuss the following key points with the patient:

KEY POINTS TO COMMUNICATE TO PATIENTS

Generalized Anxiety Disorder

1. If buspirone is prescribed, you should expect that it will take from 2–6 weeks to notice symptomatic improvement. Daily doses are required. This is not a medication that you take only as needed.

FIGURE 18

DECISION TREE FOR DIAGNOSIS AND TREATMENT OF ANXIETY

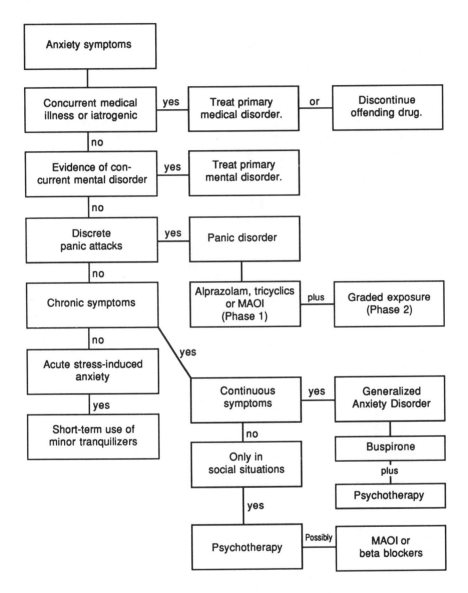

2. Often medication treatment is not enough and psychotherapy, stress management, relaxation training, and biofeedback are helpful adjuncts to medical treatment.

Stress-Related Anxiety
1. The following analogy is helpful. Pain killers can reduce suffering when you have a toothache, but at some point you must fix or pull the tooth. Likewise, minor tranquilizers do not cure people, but they temporarily reduce suffer-

ing. You must do something to alter the basic source of stress if lasting recovery is to be achieved. Minor tranquilizers are only for short-term use.
2. Do not abruptly discontinue minor tranquilizers, especially if they have been taken daily for several weeks. Cold-turkey discontinuation can result in withdrawal syndromes (many withdrawal symptoms are almost identical to symptoms of anxiety).
3. Do not drink any kind of alcohol if you are taking a minor tranquilizer.

Panic Disorder
1. There is strong evidence that panic disorder is a biochemical dysfunction, not a psychological disorder. It can often be very successfully treated with medications.
2. Medication must be taken each day. The treatment is prophylactic and not a medication that you only take as needed.
3. The medication treats *only* the panic attacks. Once these are adequately controlled, you will need to enter Phase Two of treatment (graded reexposure) to deal with anticipatory anxiety and avoidance. In many cases this is best done with the help of a therapist familiar with behavioral techniques.
4. If MAO inhibitors are used, you must understand the dietary and medication restrictions and sign a consent form.
5. If alprazolam or clonazepam are used, you must never abruptly discontinue it (medication reduction should be done gradually, generally 0.25 to 0.5 mg. per day per week).
6. If treated by tricyclics or MAOI's, it may take 2–3 weeks before you notice symptomatic changes.

Social Phobias
1. If medication is used (MAOI or beta blockers), this must be accompanied by exposure (i.e. you must be willing to enter certain social situations and test out the water).
2. Psychotherapy is probably also indicated.

Books to Recommend to Patients

The Anxiety Disease by David Sheehan, M.D., Bantam Books (1983).

Anxiety and Its Treatment by John Greist, M.D., James Jefferson, M.D., and Isaac Marks, M.D. Warner Books (1986).

---

*Also referred to as minor tranquilizers, anxiolytics, and benzodiazepines. These terms will be used interchangeably.

Chapter 5   Psychotic Disorders

DIAGNOSIS

Major Clinical Features and Differential Diagnosis

For practical purposes three major psychotic disorders are described: (1) Schizophrenia (and schizophrenic-like disorders), (2) psychotic mood disorders, and (3) psychosis associated with neurological conditions.

Before discussing differential diagnosis, let's first briefly define *psychosis*. Psychosis is not an illness; it is a symptom associated with a number of disorders. The hallmark of psychosis is impaired reality testing (impaired ability to perceive reality). The loss of contact with reality can take many forms: severe confusional states, delusions (bizarre, unrealistic thoughts), hallucinations, and marked impairment in judgment and reasoning. Having psychotic symptoms does not in itself imply a specific etiology; causes are varied. The three groups of psychotic disorders mentioned above are distinguished by the following characteristics:

1. *Schizophrenia*. Schizophrenia is generally a recurring illness; people diagnosed as schizophrenic are prone to repeated psychotic episodes. It is helpful to think about three types of schizophrenia:

   a. *Positive Symptom Schizophrenia*. This type of schizophrenia is also referred to as dopaminergic schizophrenia because of its presumed etiology: a hyperactive dopamine system. Positive symptoms are active, florid delusions and hallucinations; agitation and emotional dyscontrol. There are two subtypes:

      1. *Schizophreniform disorder* (Brief psychotic reaction). This disorder looks like schizophrenia but remits quicker and often does not recur.

      2. *Schizophrenia, per se*. This is a recurring or chronic disorder.

   b. *Negative Symptom Schizophrenia*. This is a neurodegenerative illness. Negative symptoms include: flat affect, anhedonia (inability to experience pleasure), marked social aloofness/withdrawal, and the absence of florid delusions and hallucinations. Negative symptom schizophrenia tends to have an earlier and more insidious onset. As children, these people were often seen as weird and aloof.

2. *Psychotic Mood Disorders.* Both mania and depression can present with poor reality testing and other psychotic symptoms.

3. *Psychosis Associated with Neurological Conditions.* Many acute metabolic and toxic states can result in a delirium. Head injury occasionally produces transient psychotic behavior and a number of degenerative diseases (e.g., Alzheimer's) can produce periods of agitated confusion. Detailed description of psychopharmacologic treatment of various neurological conditions is beyond the scope of this book. However, it is very important to distinguish such conditions from schizophrenia and mood disorders. A brief mental status exam can be helpful. It should include a test of short term memory, as well as tests for orientation and naming. Most neurologically based disorders that present with psychotic symptoms will also show gross impairment in recent/ short term memory and orientation. Generally, orientation and short-term memory are relatively intact in schizophrenia. Damage to Wernicke's area can occasionally result in what looks like a schizophrenic reaction (language and thinking are grossly impaired). Wernicke's patients have a terrible time naming objects; people with schizophrenia and mood disorders do not. See the *Four Minute Neurologic Exam* (in the MedMaster Series) for more hints on conducting a brief neurologic exam. Figure 19 lists medical illnesses that may produce psychotic symptoms, and Figure 20 lists medications that may result in psychotic reactions.

Figure 19

COMMON DISEASES AND DISORDERS THAT CAN CAUSE PSYCHOSIS

Addison's disease	■ Myxedema
CNS infections	■ Pancreatitis
CNS neoplasms	■ Pellagra
CNS trauma	■ Pernicious anemia
Cushing's disease	■ Porphyria
Delirium[1]	■ Systemic lupus erythematosis
Dementias[2]	■ Temporal lobe epilepsy
Folic acid deficiency	■ Thyrotoxicosis
■ Huntington's chorea	
Multiple sclerosis	

---

[1] Any number of toxic/metabolic states may result in delirium.
[2] Any number of dementing conditions (e.g., Alzheimer's disease) may result in psychotic symptoms.

Figure 20
COMMON DRUGS THAT MAY CAUSE PSYCHOSIS

■ Sympathomimetics (e.g., cocaine and "crack," a form of almost pure cocaine, many over-the-counter cold medications)

■ Antiinflammatory drugs (e.g., steroids)

■ Anticholinergic drugs (e.g., antiparkinsonian drugs)

■ Hallucinogenic drugs (e.g., LSD)

■ L-Dopa (in schizophrenic patients)

NOTE: Older persons are often on centrally acting drugs and have less ability to tolerate their toxic effects.

NOTE: The treatment of mood disorders that present with psychotic symptoms primarily involves treating the depression (tricyclics or ECT) and adding antipsychotics to control the psychotic symptoms. Since much of this has been covered previously (Chapters 2 and 3), the focus of the following sections will be on treating schizophrenia.

Target Symptons

It is helpful to subdivide schizophrenic symptoms into three categories: positive symptoms, characterological traits, and negative symptoms. (See Figure 21.)

ANTIPSYCHOTIC MEDICATION

When Do You Prescribe Antipsychotic Medication?

Although many general practitioners treat anxiety and depressive disorders, most patients presenting with psychotic symptoms should be referred to a psychiatrist. These patients are often hard to treat. Many psychotic patients can be treated on an outpatient basis; however, hospitalization is often necessary.

Antipsychotic medications (also referred to as neuroleptics or major tranquilizers) should be started when the early signs of psychosis appear, since many times a more florid psychotic episode can be averted with appropriate early intervention.

As indicated in figure 21, positive symptoms are the primary target symptoms for treatment by antipsychotic medications. Such drugs do little to affect characterological traits or negative symptoms (with some exceptions. See pages 36 and 37).

Figure 21

SCHIZOPHRENIC SYMPTOMS

POSITIVE SYMPTOMS
(Targets for Medication Treatment)

- Delusions and impaired thinking
- Hallucinations
- Confusion and impaired judgment
- Severe anxiety, agitation, and emotional dyscontrol

CHARACTEROLOGICAL
TRAITS

- Social isolation and sense of alienation
- Low self-esteem
- Social skills deficits

NEGATIVE SYMPTOMS

- Flat or blunted affect
- Poverty of thought (i.e., few or no thoughts and concrete thinking)
- Emptiness and anhedonia (no joy)
- Psychomotor retardation/inactivity
- Blunting of perception (e.g., insensitivity to pain)

Choosing a Medication

All antipsychotic medications are equally effective in their ability to reduce symptoms. The choice of medication is dictated almost exclusively by the side effect profile. For a list of antipsychotic medications, see Figure 22.

Antipsychotic medications have three primary side effects which must be taken into consideration: sedation, anticholinergic (ACH), and extrapyramidal (EPS) effects.

Before choosing a medication, assess the patient's motor state. Psychotic reactions that present with marked agitation may require more sedating drugs. Use less sedating drugs for psychoses with pronounced psychomotor retardation and withdrawal. This is a general rule of thumb, but there are exceptions.

Consider anticholinergic and EPS side effects. The most common cause for relapse is poor compliance or premature discontinuation because of unpleasant side effects. The key to successful treatment rests on how well you handle side effects.

32

Figure 22

ANTIPSYCHOTIC MEDICATIONS

GENERIC	BRAND	DOSAGE RANGE[1]	SEDATION	EPS[2]	ACH AFFECTS[3]	EQUIVALENCE[4]
Low Potency						
chlorpromazine	Thorazine	50-1500 mg	High	+ +	+ + + +	100 mg
thioridazine	Mellaril	150-800 mg	High	+	+ + + + +	100 mg
clozapine	Clozaril	300-900 mg	High	0	+ + + + +	50 mg
mesoridazine	Serentil	50-500 mg	High	+	+ + + + +	50 mg
High Potency						
molindone	Moban	20-225 mg	Low	+ + +	+ + +	10 mg
perphenazine	Trilafon	8-60 mg	Mid	+ + + +	+ +	10 mg
loxapine	Loxitane	50-250 mg	Low	+ + +	+ +	10 mg
trifluoperazine	Stelazine	10-40 mg	Low	+ + + +	+ +	5 mg
fluphenazine	Prolixin[5]	3-45 mg	Low	+ + + + +	+ +	2 mg
thiothixene	Navane	10-60 mg	Low	+ + + +	+ +	5 mg
haloperidol	Haldol[5]	2-40 mg	Low	+ + + + +	+	2 mg
pimozide	Orap	1-10 mg	Low	+ + + + +	+	2 mg

(1) Usual daily oral dosage.
(2) Acute: Parkinson's dystonias, akathesia. Does not reflect risk for tardive dyskinesia. All neuroleptics may cause tardive dyskinesia, except clozapine.
(3) Anticholinergic Side Effects: dry mouth, constipation, urinary retention, and blurry vision.
(4) Dose required to achieve efficacy of 100 mg chlorpromazine.
(5) Available in time-released IM format.

Extrapyramidal Side Effects. There are four classes of EPS:
1. *Parkinson-like Side Effects.* These include muscular rigidity, flat affect (mask-like facial expression), tremor, bradykinesia (slowed motor responses). These symptoms need to be distinguished from the flat affect and withdrawal often seen as primary symptoms of schizophrenia. Parkinson-like side effects are often diminished by the administration of anticholinergic agents (e.g., benzotropine, trihexylphenidyl, or amantadine).
2. *Akathisia.* This is an uncontrolled sense of inner restlessness. Akathisia must be distinguished from anxiety. Often, a physician may mistake it for anxiety and increase the dose of antipsychotic, only to see a worsening of the restlessness. Akathisia can be partially alleviated by anticholinergic agents. Other drugs, however, are often more successful. These include diphenhydramine, propranolol, or minor tranquilizers, such as lorazepam.
3. *Acute Dystonias.* These are muscle spasms and prolonged muscular contractions, usually of the head and neck. These can be resolved quickly with intramuscular anticholinergic agents, or treated prophylactically with oral anticholinergics.
4. *Tardive Dyskinesia (TD).* TD is generally a late onset EPS. This is a very serious and often irreversible effect of antipsychotic medication treatment. It

affects about one out of 25 people treated for a period of one year, and by seven years of continuous treatment, it affects one in four. Symptoms include involuntary sucking and smacking movements of the mouth and lips, and can include chorea in the trunk and extremities. Although various drugs have been used to reduce TD symptoms (e.g., baclofen, sodium valporate, lecithin, and benzodiazepines), there is no true cure. Treatment starts with stopping the medication. Initial worsening of the dyskinesia is expected, as the drug not only causes the syndrome but also tends to mask it. Be patient, for months if necessary, and TD will often remit. But control of severe psychosis usually outweighs the problem of TD. All patients receiving antipsychotics *must* sign an informed consent form which explains the risks of TD.

Anticholinergic Side Effects. These are the same as described in Chapter 2 on depression.

The Relationship Between Side Effects. Anticholinergic agents reduce EPS. You may coadminister neuroleptics and anticholinergics, or you may use certain antipsychotics which have anticholinergic metabolites. The chart below is a simple way to remember how the various side effects relate to one another.

DRUG CLASSES		SIDE EFFECTS	
(See Figure 22)	Sedation	ACH	EPS
Low Potency	High	High	Low
High Potency	Low	Low	High
Please see Figure 22 for a more detailed outline of antipsychotic side effects.			

Several potentially serious additional side effects can occur with antipsychotic medications, including agranulocytosis, impaired temperature regulations and thus increased risk of heat stroke, and neuroleptic malignant syndrome (a very rare syndrome that presents with fever, extrapyramidal rigidity, severe autonomic dysfunction and in some cases death. For a detailed review of this syndrome, see Pearlman, 1986). For these reasons, treatment of psychotic disorders is often more appropriately carried out by a psychiatrist.

Prescribing Treatment and What to Expect

Antipsychotic medications are generally started at low to moderate doses and titrated up until there is reduction in the more disruptive aspects of the psychotic reaction, e.g., agitation. (NOTE: Some clinicians recommend "rapid neuroleptization," i.e., very high initial doses of neuroleptics. This treatment approach is controversial). Divided doses may be helpful initially; however, after a few days, a switch to a once-a-day bedtime dose is advisable. Dosage ranges are extremely broad and vary considerably from patient to patient. In outpatient practice, an initial starting dose might be haloperidol 2mg./day or with chlorpromazine, 100mg./day. Inpatients are often treated at higher initial doses. See Figure 22 for dosage ranges. Antipsychotic medications must be taken each day.

Symptomatic improvement initially is seen as a decrease in arousal, emotional dyscontrol, and agitation. Poor reality testing, hallucinations, and disordered thinking may take much longer to respond. In many chronic schizophrenics, these latter symptoms may take a number of weeks to respond.

Assuming a good response, how long do you continue to treat? If the psychotic episode is a first episode, the rule of thumb is to decrease to a maintenance dose and continue to treat for one year. If the episode is a repeated episode, will probably be best to treat for two to three years before a medication-free trial is initiated. Always, owing to the risk of TD, one should treat at the lowest possible dose that provides symptomatic relief.

Figure 23

DECISION TREE FOR DIAGNOSIS AND TREATMENT OF PSYCHOSIS

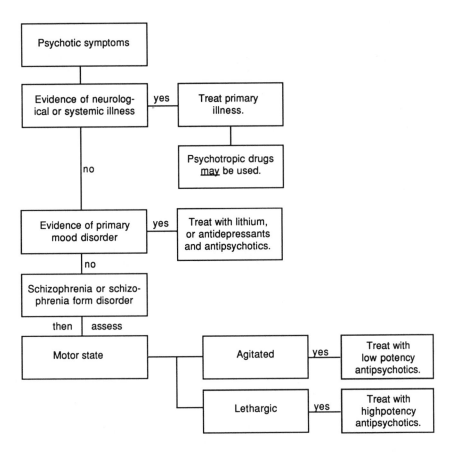

KEY POINTS TO COMMUNICATE TO PATIENTS

1. It is important to describe side effects to patients, especially akathisia. This side effect can be extremely unpleasant, yet often it is not spontaneously reported by patients. If it occurs and is not treated, this will greatly increase the risk of noncompliance, as well as increasing the patient's suffering. So tell patients, "You may notice an inner feeling of restlessness or nervousness. If you do, please tell me. Do not just discontinue the medication. Most side effects can be treated."

2. Schizophrenia is a relapsing disorder and it is extremely important to keep taking medication even if things seem fine. Premature discontinuation is the primary cause of relapse.

3. The total length of treatment is likely to be at least one year and often longer for more chronic schizophrenia.

4. Antipsychotic medications are not addictive.

5. You should avoid prolonged exposure to high temperatures and sunlight (some antipsychotics have photosensitivity as a side effect).

6. Avoid amphetamines, cocaine, and L-Dopa because these drugs always exacerbate psychoses.

7. You and your relatives need to know about the risk of TD (and sign appropriate consent forms).

Treatment-Resistant Schizophrenic Disorders

There are three main reasons why schizophrenic patients may not respond to antipsychotic medication:

1. *Poor compliance*. Often this is due to the unpleasant side effects. Many times patient education and proper medical management of side effects resolve the problem. Sometimes, patients simply forget to take their medication. In such cases, treatment with time-released intramuscular forms of antipsychotics can be helpful.

2. *Inadequate doses*. Blood levels can be monitored and doses increased as indicated.

3. So-called negative symptom schizophrenics may have a different underlying pathophysiology and often do not respond well to traditional antipsychotics. These patients are hard to treat. Some authors have suggested the use of anticholinergics or benzodiazepines to treat these patients, but at this point truly successful treatments are not available.

Two antipsychotic medications have shown promise in treating the negative (as well as positive) symptoms of schizophrenia. The first is clozapine (brand name Clozaril). Clozapine became available in the United States in early 1990. This medication is considered to be an atypical antipsychotic agent; its pharmacologic profile is different than other existing antipsychotics. The first important feature is that initial trials show it to be effective in treating many schizophrenic patients who have failed to respond to standard antipsychotic drugs. This includes a number of patients that presented with negative symptoms (as well as other treatment-resistant schizophrenics). The second important and unique feature is the virtual lack of acute extrapyramidal symptoms and few reported cases of tardive dyskinesia. This medication does have two significant potential side effects: (1) The incidence of clozapine-induced agranulocytosis (a potentially fatal blood dyscrasia) is between 1 and 2%, as compared to the incidence seen in other antipsychotics (about 0.1%). This problem, however, is proving to be avoidable through a mandatory hematological monitoring program (weekly medication dispensing occurs only if the patient's white blood cell count is normal). Since implementing this program, there have been no fatalities in the 15 cases of clozapine-related agranulocytosis reported in the United States. If there is a low WBC count, medication is immediately discontinued and, to date, all such cases have been reversible. (2) A second troublesome side effect is a fairly high incidence of seizures (about 1–2% at low doses and 5% at higher doses). Despite these problematic features, clozapine appears to represent an important breakthrough in the management of otherwise treatment-resistant schizophrenic disorders.

A second medication, soon to be released, which appears to target both positive and negative symptoms is risperidone.

Books to Recommend to Patients and Their Families

Surviving Schizophrenia: A Family Manual by E. Fuller Torrey, M.D., Harper and Row Publishers (1983).

Chapter 6   Miscellaneous Disorders

In this final chapter we would like to briefly discuss a couple of additional disorders for which psychotropic medications can be useful.

Obsessive-Compulsive Disorder

Major Clinical Features

The major features of this disorder are recurring obsessions (persistent, intrusive, troublesome thoughts or impulses that are recognized by the patient as senseless) and/or compulsions (repetitive behaviors or rituals enacted in response to an obsession, e.g. repeatedly checking to see if doors are locked, compulsive hand washing, or counting). In order to meet the criteria for obsessive compulsive disorder, the obsessions and/or compulsions must create significant distress or be time consuming enough to interfere with normal routines (APA, 1987).

Medication Treatment

| *NAME* | | | | |
Generic	Brand	Dose Range	Sedation	ACH Effects
clomipramine	Anafranil	150–300 mg	Hi	Hi
fluoxetine	Prozac[1]	20–80 mg	Low	None
sertraline	Zoloft[1]	50–200 mg	Low	None
paroxetine	Paxil	20–50 mg	Low	None

[1]often higher doses are required to control obsessive-compulsive symptoms than the doses generally used to treat depression.

Books To Recommend To Patients and Their Families

Obsessive-Compulsive
Rapoport, J. L. (1989). *The Boy Who Couldn't Stop Washing.* Signet: New York.

Borderline Personality Disorder

Major Clinical Features

Borderline personality disorders constitute a very heterogeneous group of individuals that suffer from long-term emotional instability. As a group they are characterized by the following features: a pattern of chaotic, unstable relationships, significant emotional lability, impulsiveness (e.g. self-mutilation, suicide attempts, substance abuse, very poor frustration tolerance, sexual promiscuity), anger control problems (e.g. pronounced irritability, temper tantrums, etc.), a tendency to develop significant bouts of anxiety and depression, and chronic feelings of emptiness. Some borderline patients can develop transient psychotic symptoms (that usually remit within hours to days). These patients are prone to any number of major psychiatric syndromes in addition to what is a very stable, chronic pattern of maladaptive functioning in life.

Medication Treatment

Although there may be some underlying biologic cause in some of these patients, it is generally felt that the basic disorder is an outgrowth of significant early, maladaptive psychological development. Psychotropic medications in no way treat the basic personality disorder, however, medications can be used to treat particular target symptoms. The literature is sparce on the pharmacologic treatment of borderline disorders. However, clinical case reports and a handful of empirical studies are beginning to provide some helpful guidelines for pharmacologic treatment.

Not all borderline patients are alike, and for treatment purposes, the following subgroups can be delineated to provide guidelines for choosing medications. The subgroups are defined by the presence of a dominant symptom picture.

SUB-GROUPS	DRUGS OF CHOICE
1. Impulsivity/Anger Control Problems	Serotonergic anti-depressants, e.g. fluoxetine, sertraline
2. Schizotypal (peculiar thinking, transient psychosis)	Low doses of anti-psychotic medications e.g. 1 mg. haloperidol, 25–50 mg thioridazine
3. Extreme sensitivity to rejection/ being alone	MAO inhibitors; serotonergic anti-depressants

Note: investigators to date have found that minor tranquilizers generally are not indicated in the treatment of borderline personality disorder. These patients often experience an increased degree of emotional dyscontrol/disinhibition with minor tranquilizers, and are at high risk for abusing such drugs.

For more information, the reader is referred to two review articles:

Cowdry, R. W. and Gardner, D. L. (1988). "Pharmacotherapy of Borderline Personality Disorder." *Archives of General Psychiatry,* Vol. 45, p. 111–119.

Cornelius, J. R., et. al. (1991). "A Preliminary Trial of Fluoxetine in Refractory Borderline Patients." *Journal of Clinical Psychopharmacology,* Vol. 11, No. 2, p. 116–120.

Books To Recommend To Patients and Their Families

Borderline Personality Disorder
Kreisman J., and Krauss, H. (1989). *I Hate You—Don't Leave Me: Understanding Borderline Personality Disorder.* Price Stern: New York.

Appendix A
History and Personal Data Questionnaire

Date:_____

Name: _____ Date of birth: _____ Age:____

Main reason for seeking help at this time: _____
_____
_____

Current Problems or Symptoms

Please read each item below and determine which statement is true for you. Then, place an "X" in the appropriate box to indicate how often you feel the statement applies to you during the past month.

Be sure to rate every item.   *Example:*

	None or a little of the time	Some of the time	Most or all of the time
1. I feel sad.		X	

DURING THE PAST MONTH	None or a little of the time	Some of the time	Most or all of the time
A 1. Wake up at night or in the early morning and unable to return to sleep			
2. Very restless sleep			
3. Loss of energy			
4. Decreased sex drive			
5. Unable to enjoy life; have lost a zest for life			
6. Have withdrawn from others			
7. Strong thoughts about suicide			
8. Loss of appetite			
9. Memory problem, forgetfulness, poor concentration			
10. Weight loss (How much in past month? ____lbs) Weight gain (How much in past month? ____lbs) Have you been trying to diet? ❏ Yes ❏ No			

Appendix A
History and Personal Data Questionnaire, Cont'd.

	DURING THE PAST MONTH	None or a little of the time	Some of the time	Most or all of the time
B 11.	Decreased need for sleep			
12.	Increased sex drive			
13.	Increased energy			
14.	So happy that people describe me as "manic"			
C 15.	Can't get to sleep			
16.	Sudden episodes of nervousness or panic			
17.	Fear of losing self-control			
18.	Palpitations or rapid heart beat			
19.	Shortness of breath			
D 20.	Strange or unusual thoughts			
21.	Hallucinations, hear voices, or see things that aren't there			
22.	Very peculiar experiences			
E 23.	Ready to explode			
24.	Thoughts about harming someone			
25.	Excessive use of alcohol/drugs			

Previous Treatment For Emotional Problems

Year	Problem	Therapist/Location	Hospitalization or Medical Treatment

All Current Medications	Dosage	Schedule	Doctor

Medical Information
Have you ever been diagnosed as having the following? (Please check all that apply to you.)

- ❑ Heart trouble
- ❑ Thyroid disease
- ❑ Diabetes
- ❑ Vascular (circulation) disease
- ❑ Seizure disorder
- ❑ High blood pressure
- ❑ Ulcers
- ❑ Head injury

Thank You.

Appendix B

SPECIAL CAUTIONS WHEN TAKING MAO INHIBITORS

A Patient Hand-Out

MAO Inhibitors can be very safe and effective antidepressant medications. However, certain foods and drugs must be avoided while taking MAO Inhibitors. Mixing MAO Inhibitors with the following drugs/foods can cause a serious rise in blood pressure.

FOODS TO AVOID

Cheese (Philadelphia cream cheese and cottage cheese are OK.)
Chicken liver and beef liver
Yeast preparations (avoid Brewer's yeast, powdered and caked yeast as sold in health food stores, Bakery yeast is OK.)
Fava or broad beans
Herring (pickled or kippered)
Beer, sherry, ale, red wine, liqueurs
Canned figs
Protein extracts (found in some dried soups, soup cubes, and commercial gravies)
Certain meat products; bologna, salami, pepperoni, Spam

AVOID EXCESSIVE AMOUNTS OF THESE FOODS

Yogurt and/or sour cream
Ripe avocados and guacamole
Chocolate and/or caffeine
White wine and liquors

MEDICATIONS TO AVOID

Stimulant drugs (amphetamines, dexadrine, benzedine, methedrine, methylphenidate)
Diet pills
Cocaine, "crack"
Cold preparations, including over-the-counter products which contain decongestants (e.g., Sudafed, Contac, etc.). Antihistamines and aspirin are OK.
Nasal sprays

- Adrenalin (Make sure that your dentist knows you are taking MAO Inhibitors because many local anesthetics contain adrenalin.)
- Please talk with your physician before taking any new medications (prescription or over-the-counter.)

SYMPTOMS OF DRUG OR FOOD INTERACTION

While taking MAO Inhibitors, if you ever experience the following symptoms, please contact your physician or an emergency room immediately.

- Severe headache
- Excessive perspiration
- Lightheadedness
- Vomiting
- Increased heart rate

I have read and understand the above precautions.

Patient's Name _____Date_____
Signature

References

1. American Psychiatric Association (1987) *Diagnostic and Statistical Manual of Mental Disorders—III—Revised* (DSM-III-R). APA, Washington, DC.

2. Baldessarini, R. J. and Cole, J. O. (1988) "Chemotherapy" in *The New Harvard Guide to Psychiatry*, edited by A. M. Nicholi, Harvard University Press, Cambridge, Mass.

3. Goldberg, Stephen (1987) *The Four-Minute Neurologic Exam*, MedMaster, Inc., Miami.

4. Nicholi, A. M. (ed.) (1988) *The New Harvard Guide to Psychiatry*, Harvard University Press, Cambridge, Mass.

5. Unlenhuth, E. H., DeWit, H., Balter, M. B., Johanson, C. E. and Mellinger, G. D. (1988) "Risks and benefits of long term benzodiazepine use." *Journal of Clinical Psychopharmacology*, 8:161–167.

6. Pearlman, C. A. (1986) "Neuroleptic malignant syndrome: A review of the literature." *Journal of Clinical Psychopharmacology,* 6:257–273.